The Voices of Autoimmune Arthritis

The Voices of Autoimmune Arthritis

Edited by Kahlianna Manriquez

Authors

Kahlianna Manriquez

Tami Brown

Lindsey McBee

Therese Humphrey

Cindy Gilchrist

Lorna K

Tara Manriquez

Introduction

Kahlianna Manriquez

I thought of this book when I had finished reading an anthology book. I wanted to publish another book, but I did not have an idea for a full book and the anthology I just read gave me an idea why don't I put together an anthology. The next part was to think of a theme for the anthology. My mom (Tara Manriquez) was writing a blog to spread the word about Rheumatoid Arthritis, so I thought why don't I collect peoples stories of their autoimmune arthritis. This new idea could help spread the word and raise money to help one of the charities that supports autoimmune arthritis. That is how we ended up with *The Voices of Autoimmune Arthritis*.

Tami Brown

I had always been such an active, athletic woman that I didn't really notice what was going on at first, except that my feet hurt more by the end of the day, but I guess I was thinking it had to do with my shoes or from my daily runs. This was around 1998, while I was living in Michigan and working as the Executive Secretary to the Chief of Police of my town's police department. It was so bad I actually brought a pair of fuzzy slippers to work with me, so I could take off my street shoes and wear my slippers under my desk! By the end of 1999, I couldn't ignore it anymore. My toes were red and swollen and they'd become deformed, with the big toes turned inward 90 degrees and some toes on top of others. I'd been an avid runner all my life (5-6 miles every day), so the orthopedic surgeon I saw just blamed it on my running; although he was so shocked to see how much arthritis damage there was in my feet at the age of 39 that he actually called in his partners to view my x-rays and my feet! After 2 surgeries on one foot and 1 surgery on the other (in 1999 and 2000), where surgical rods and pins were permanently inserted, bone was cut out, and tendons were snipped to repair the damage, I was sent on my way and told there would be no more running for me. No one even thought about the possibility of RA.

Next I found out I had endometriosis and was filled with fibroids and ovarian cysts (in 2001) and required surgery for that. After that, I kept getting one infection after another – kidneys, sinuses, bladder - and I even had a bout of kidney stones. I remember now that my internal medicine doc at the time was getting tired of pumping me with antibiotics, and he said I should probably be checked for autoimmune illness, but at the time I had no idea what that was. He told me the test came back negative so I never gave it a second thought.

Shortly after that, I got an offer for a new job closer to my parents in Indiana, and I moved. That meant starting over with a new doctor.

For another year or more I continued to suffer from recurring infections and kidney stones and pancreatitis, but in between the infections, other symptoms started to surface. I started getting drenching night sweats, rashes after being out in the sun, fevers that would come and go and days where I'd just feel like I had the flu – nausea and fatigue that was so off the charts that I was calling off sick from work more and more often. I remember there were several occasions that I actually fell asleep at the wheel driving to and from work. I'm amazed I didn't kill myself (or someone else) during that period, as I had a 40 minute commute each way. Then I started getting swelling in my finger joints along with redness and heat on the large finger joints. At this point, late 2003 at the age of 43, my new internist also said, "We need to test you for autoimmune illness!" This time my RF factor came back positive, so she sent me off to a rheumatologist. Several months later, when I was finally get in to see a rheumatologist in early 2004, he diagnosed me with RA and possible lupus (I still have "crossover" symptoms and although my ANA remains positive, I have enough clinical criteria to diagnose, so my doctor is treating me for lupus as well. Since my initial diagnosis I have also had the diagnosis of Sjogren's Syndrome and Raynaud's Phenomenon added to my roster, and I'd already had Hashimoto's Thyroiditis which was diagnosed way back in 1994 – even BEFORE my foot surgeries!). My rheumatologist told me that based on my blood work and the damage observed in my joint x-rays, as well as the history of symptoms we were able to now piece together over the years, I had likely had the disease for at least years.

Five years later I was no longer able to continue working. I was completely unprepared for this eventuality. My body may have been unable to keep up with the physical demands, but not my heart or my mind. I made several valiant efforts to try part-time jobs and work-at-home jobs, but none of them worked out. We also tried various medication combinations, but still, none were able to stabilize me well enough to allow me to remain employed. According to my rheumatologist, by the time my disease was finally diagnosed, it was "running like a freight train", and it was too aggressive for the medications to stabilize it both at that level of activity and level of stress, and there was too much irreversible damage exacerbating the problems.

Diagnosis autoimmune arthritis illnesses, though improving, is still taking far too long, and patients are suffering for it; by way of unnecessary pain, permanent joint damage and/or disability. Education and awareness surrounding these diseases MUST be increased. Both patients and physicians must understand that oftentimes symptoms arrive before all the necessary inflammatory markers that would allow for an exact diagnosis show up in the blood, but that doesn't mean that treatment must wait as well. A sero-negative patient who is symptomatic, especially if there are signs of joint damage, needs to be referred to a rheumatologist, and early and aggressive treatment should be started in order to prevent permanent joint damage, disability, or even death.

Lindsey McBee

For 22 years I wasn't the healthiest person but didn't have any major medical issues. Then one night I went to bed and when I woke up my joints were stiff and swollen. My doctors moved quickly to diagnose the problem and within the year, my rheumatologist had confirmed a diagnosis of sero-negative, ANA positive Rheumatoid Arthritis. Immediately I began aggressive treatment to help manage my symptoms and slowly reduce the amount of steroids I had to take. Being diagnosed with RA, trying to live with RA, and managing the side-effects of the medication were difficult for me but were even more difficult for my husband. We had only been married for 2 years when I was diagnosed and he wasn't prepared to have a wife with a chronic disease. After my diagnosis I began to have circulatory, eye, and thyroid problems that were all related to RA. At 24 I made the decision to have a hysterectomy due to ongoing health problems. With everything going on, I wasn't the same person that my husband had married and he began to resent me. By the time I was 26 the marriage was over. He couldn't handle living with someone who had severe RA and I couldn't continue to live with someone who hated me for having RA.

Despite my diagnosis, the medical complications, and my divorce, I returned to college; I earned my B.S. in Rehabilitation Studies and soon will graduate with my M.S. in Behavior Analysis (hopefully August of 2014). This journey hasn't been easy, I don't know if I will be able to work full-time upon graduation, and I don't know how I will continue to pay for my healthcare. However, with the amazing support of my family, being able to work with the amazing people at IFAA, and a will to fight...I refuse to let my diagnose define me. RA can happen to anyone and it doesn't do anyone any good to wallow in sorrow or self-pity. In the past year my disease has progressed which has caused some complications in my graduate studies but I will graduate and I will do something to help those less fortunate than me. It has been over 7 years since I was diagnosed and almost 8 years since symptoms began but I have continued to work, finish my education, and work with others.

This biggest tool in my arsenal to manage the day to day living of RA has been humor. I laugh at the things that I can't control and try to find humor during my ongoing infusions by joking with the nurses and other patients. Sometimes I find it is good to cry but that is a rare occasion. Humor has been the best medicine for me. I take all the pills the doctor prescribes, endure the infusions and increasing medication dose, I work through the pain, and I always try to smile. I don't believe RA defines me nor do I believe RA has swallowed me whole. There will always be bad days but those bad days are often followed by awesome days. We have to remember that you have to have a little rain in order to have a few rainbows.

Therese Humphrey

It was July 1986, I was newly married at the time, age 26, when I was diagnosed with Rheumatoid Arthritis. I had been a very active, young, vibrant woman when a sudden onset of swollen, painful knees and feet happened within days, leaving me unable to walk. My husband within a month of my diagnosis started doing everything for me. He had to help dress me, carry me up and down the stairs and even help me to the toilet. I was sure I was going to die. I was exhausted all of the time and was in constant pain. Looking back, I really think he resented me for it and never fully understood what was happening…but then again, neither did I.

I felt alone and depressed, with no where & no one to turn to…but somehow, I never gave up hope. Looking back I realize how strong I really was- I would hide my pain from others, never complaining to them mainly because I had no idea what was happening to my body and thought if I would pretend it wasn't happening-it would just go away.

Friends and even some family didn't understand what it meant for me to have an "autoimmune" arthritis, especially since so many just thought it was "just arthritis", not ever realizing it affects the entire body not "just joints."

I was crying one day because I was in so much pain and instead of being comforted by my husband, he told me to stop crying, pull myself together and take more of my medicine. At that time, I was taking high doses of aspirin. Needless to say, after several years of going to many Rheumatologist appointments by myself, crying at night alone…my marriage came to an end.

I was told by my Rheumatologist after a couple years of never ending medication trial and errors, that I would more than likely, be in a wheelchair within 10 years. I am absolutely convinced that if it had not been for the new FDA approved Biologic Enbrel that came out in 1998, an anti-TNF injection, I would have been wheelchair bound right now. I was still in pain everyday but I was able to live a lot more of a normal life. "I had a wonderful career," as a Registered Nurse in the Intensive Care Unit. However, due to the persistent inflammation of RA & not having the proper treatment at that time to stop the progression, my career I loved ended far earlier than I had planned. I was disabled. After battling the disease for 10 yrs., RA caused some of my joints to be totally destroyed with bone erosion & destruction of cartilage leaving me with complete loss of joint integrity in both wrists, one of my ankles and both feet. At present, I have had reconstructive surgery on both my feet. Having an autoimmune arthritis disease can affect each and everyone of us differently depending on many influences ; from medication efficacy to coping skills on dealing with pain, joints affected, fatigue and other symptoms that can occur.

Our challenges seem to change on a daily basis due to the fact that Rheumatoid Autoimmune Arthritis symptoms can come and go and can be very unpredictable. Today I am on a combination treatment of Humira (Biologic injection) and Methotrexate. I still experience pain and I still have flare ups, but overtime, I have learned to deal with these when they happen. Not everyone is as lucky as me, not everyone responds to treatments as well as I have. There is so much more that is still not understood about RA. Treatments are always improving but still there is no cure. The most valuable aspect I have gained with this diagnosis, is that I have met thousands of truly inspirational people fighting the same battle of this invisible chronic disease via social media. I try my best to help others struggling with similar challenges brought on by RA & give them hope to never give up the fight. In doing so, I have found that my own burden of feeling alone is no longer and for that I am grateful.

I micromanage my life everyday- There are some things that I cannot do, however, I choose to focus on all the things I "can do."

My RA story: Cindy Gilchrist age 50

I welcome the opportunity to share my Rheumatoid Arthritis experience. I am not a writer and everyone has a story. I prefer to call RA Rheumatoid Autoimmune Disease.   So many people assume it is 'just arthritis". Relatively new to the world of autoimmune disorders with just two and half years under my belt, I remain grateful I was not struck down at an earlier age as so many others have been. My story will be brief and in no way unique. What it was like, what happened and what is like today.

Yes, I had the good life prior to diagnosis. I am glad I did the all the vacations and enjoyed wide range of friends and activities. I did not miss a thing. In 2011, I had just moved back to home to Pittsburgh PA after living in Wisconsin for 6 years enduring a bad marriage and a worse divorce.   Just thrilled to be home again, familiar territory, family and renewing old friendships. I had scored a top notch account executive sales position with a well-known technology company.   I could barely believe my good fortune, someone pinch me.   I was making plans. With a good cash flow, I was surfing the internet weekly to purchase a home.   I began dating and found love with a fabulous man I adored and could not seem to spend enough time with.

The stars had finally aligned for me in my perception. I was 47 and it felt like a brand new exciting life was beginning. Planning, saving money, and dreams and hopes were plentiful for my future. Having come through many hard times but my soul felt a strong sense of peace and love. Opportunities were choices and not something I had to wait for to come my way.   As some snapshots of time are, that one was all too brief.

What happened? Wow, heavy fatigue set in. I began questioning why I was sleeping so much and seemingly not by choice. My hands became so sore. I purchased wrist guards, assuming carpal tunnel from decades of computer use. My shoulders ached; it must be the job, slugging my luggage and equipment across my sales territory. My primary care doctor agreed. Nothing unusual in the regular blood screen. I was advised to slow down, reduce stress, and take vitamins and balm for my shoulder. I heard the cliché of "you are getting older" Cindy. I left the doctor's office a few times thinking this not me, I feel sick, too sick.

My symptoms continued to worsen. I woke up one day in such pain; I knew something was happening to my whole body and not just parts. Suddenly I thought of my grandfather. My grandfather had RA and had endured so much prior to his death from RA. My brother was suffering with Psoriatic Arthritis. A 45 year old cousin in a nursing home with MS. Given my family medical history, it is hard to believe I had never considered this could be possible. I returned to the primary care doctor and specifically asked for an RA blood test! He was quite skeptical as my issues were not visible or textbook, I insisted. "The call" came shortly afterward to book an appointment with a rheumatologist as soon as possible. The blood work was positive. RA factor and SED Rate quite high. I remember the call as most of us probably do. My heart just sank. No! No! I knew RA from the view of a child, watching my grandfather in desperate pain, mangled more than crippled, and passing on early in his life. I must have googled RA every day waiting for my new Rheumatologist doctor visit. I was so frightened and fear is still a part of my life today.

I began short term disability from work as a treatment path designed for the incurable degenerative disease.   DMARD's, biologics, eventually two rounds at chemo treatment of Rituximab. Alas, I am in 30% of unresponsive patients depending on the statistics that are published. I am not surprised. I felt it in my heart and soul, as no other family member responded to medical intervention.

Mentally and physically rising and falling with each medication regime. What a draining experience. It is like getting by a train, but no one can tell. The ever spinning questions. Will this drug, give me my old life back? Can I get back to my career? I cannot imagine not working, what will I do without income? I have responsibilities and mounting medical bills. A life. More diagnoses seem to flood in. Sjogrens, Lupus syndrome, Raynaud's disease, edema, vasculitis, carpal tunnel syndrome, disc degeneration, lumbar facet joint disease.

I eventually went from my employer's short term disability, to no income then to SSDI. I waited almost two years before applying for SSDI. Foolish even stupid in hindsight. I just could not attach the word disabled to myself.   I had never realized how much of my personal identity was my career, work, and my life until I lost it almost as swiftly as a car accident. Taught as a young child, that if you work hard, you will always be able to make your own choices and life decisions.   It was my mantra.   Disabled? One word packing the punch of a professional boxer.   The stigma and my own perception were negative.   Not to mention, that those around me undermined what RA was all about.   They did not understand my "trauma" and thought is drama.

My life became akin to the country music I love.   The losses mounted quickly. First the lucrative career compounded with large medical bills, the steady decline of physical abilities, the loss of choices, a despairing decision to give up my residence. I couldn't manage it physically or financially. Disposing of once treasured possessions to fit into one bedroom at my parents' home. Shortly after the move, came the break up with my boyfriend, he said he did not see a future with me. The heart break is my final loss. Can I cope without this love in my life? I have no choice and I have hit the bottom.

What is it like today? I work daily on my own self maintenance. Medications, ice packs, heating pad, sleeping, seeing many specialists, medical bills, regular shrink visits. Life is all about just trying to manage my physical condition du jour.

Gaining recognition that this is the first thing in my life I will not conquer. I have risen above many experiences in the past. A battle with alcoholism, a painful miscarriage, three divorces, and the deaths of loved ones. Unlike previous life events, RA will not pass or get better with time. It is still a hard concept for me to grasp. I was raised as a strong independent Christian woman. We conquer, we pray and we heal and rise again.

I must accept and continually find new coping mechanisms to deal with the twists and turns on this road.

We call this one of the invisible diseases. Outwardly appearing "normal" unless I am using my cane and braces. I must learn to accept that no one other than my fellow RA friends will understand the depth and breadth of this affliction. Ongoing psychology therapy is a must. Friends, acquaintances and even family members can still give me the skeptical eye. Is she really as sick as she says? She doesn't look ill? I saw her out last week. I only speak for myself however we share the commonality of not receiving any validation. It is beyond frustrating.

Why can't people see? Even those closest to me? People that have known me for decades? I want to plead with them, tell them I feel like I am dying inside, please help me. The medical community spells out incurable. Incurable is now a feeling, not a word. I can feel this cursing (yes cursing and coursing) through my veins, eating away like that old Pac man video game. Doctors shrug their shoulders too often and look away. When do you go to the hospital? Not for fever, chills, even chest pain (arthritis of chest joints), not swelling (all normal), not for strange growths on my body (RA Cysts), not for rashes or a racing heart due to pain. Three trips to urgent care taught me that lesson.

I live my life in moments of normality, hopefully a few hours, rarely a whole day. I do not have cancer yet I take chemo medication in pill form each week. My hair has thinned; my skin is covered in various rashes and lesions. I use makeup to cover and not just my face any longer. Taking a shower, blow drying my hair and applying makeup takes twice as long and frequently need to rest afterwards before heading out the door.

I can succumb to the pity party syndrome. I still grieve the loss of my old life as one would the death of a loved one. In therapy, we discuss serious issues including suicidal idealization. How long do I really want to live? Fears over my declining quality of life. Planning of activities, never knowing how my body will be on that day. Specific activities are no longer in my list of choices, concerts, sporting events, movie theatres and or anything that requires a longer walk or has uncomfortable seating. Dating now seems like a ludacris. The average person cannot seem to perceive a partially bed ridden existence when I appear outwardly presentable. I recently had a serious conversation with a new man I have had several outings with. He mentioned taking walks in the spring? I cannot "stroll" anywhere. Walking now means to a destination, and not for pleasure. Things always seem far away to me now. The back of a store, the distance to a front door, the now ominous stairs. I will not be strolling along the beautiful skyline where he lives or walk the flea markets he enjoys. I am no longer girlfriend material. I can only hope to bring a smile, laughter and a nice evening; however I cannot be an active participant in someone else's life. Heck, I am rarely a participant in my own life.

I work on gratitude. I make gratitude lists. I pray constantly. Praise God when I have attended an event and enjoyed myself. A normal activity is worthy of a verbal thank you to the Lord. I now appreciate the smallest of gestures. A kind word of genuine understanding. My young nieces. Hugs from loved ones. A warm climate quick trip. I love the solitude of the quiet ocean waves. My feet in the sand, sun on my face and the spectacular view of the ocean. Healing power of dipping into warm sea waters. I need to load up on prednisone (I have some awful side effects) to go. Someday I will not be able to.

I am so very grateful for loving two loving parents that took me into their home after leaving some 25 years ago. The love of the people that have stayed in my life despite my frequent depression and physical condition. RA surely clears the crowd. The blessing of a new friend that will not compare the old Cindy to the Cindy with RA. A purposeful lowering of expectations creates joy in the unexpected moments. Communicating with my RA Facebook friends that share their experiences validating I am not crazy but have the same crazy symptoms we all share.

I am committed to investing my time as wisely as I used to manage my finances. I seem to have so little time when I feel well; I must take immediate advantage to catch up on the menial tasks such as laundry and the mail.

I have always been a woman of faith, raised by strong Christian women. My faith can falter with the prognosis, acceptance of the drastic life changes and long term outlook, faith carries me along. My prayer life has changed as well. I pray for strength to endure my autoimmune disorders with grace and dignity. I know God is with me. I pray to see a lighted path ahead, one day at time. Jeremiah 29: God has amazing plans for you. We live one day at a time. When ill, we cope. When moments of ability come, we grab it. My wise beloved grandmother had been right along, when you have your health you have everything you need.

Lorna K

Why me? Why not me? I would rather it be me than my husband, my children, my grandchildren or you!

There are millions of people all over the world diagnosed everyday with an Autoimmune Arthritis Disease such as Rheumatoid Arthritis, Lupus, Sjogren's Syndrome, Juvenile Arthritis, just to name a few.

These diseases don't discriminate, they attack the young, the old, the rich, the poor, the exact cause is not yet known. There is no cure, although I believe they are a lot closer to one than when I was diagnosed back in 1988.

We look fine most of the time on the outside but on the inside our immune systems are hard at work attacking our organs causing swelling, fatigue, joint pain, fevers, I could go on forever with the symptoms I have dealt with over the past 25+ years.

I don't remember a time when I felt 100% healthy, as a child I remember curling up in a ball on the floor screaming bloody murder night after night. In those days they called it "growing pains." Eventually they stopped but at the time it was pure hell! I wouldn't wish that kind of pain on anybody.

Then came my teenager years, people thought I was lazy all I wanted to do was sleep. I was always tired ! When my friends were out running around partying I was at home in bed asleep. I slept at school, at dinner pretty much everywhere.

Somehow I managed to make it through school, get married give birth to my two children not without life threatening complications.

After that life consisted of going to work, going home, cooking, cleaning, going back to work, sleeping when I could find the time. I was always on the go. During that period in my life I felt great!

Then one night at work my arm wouldn't move it it locked up, I was sent to the emergency room to get it looked at. I was diagnosed with Tendonitis. I was sent home with orders to rest, ice it and to take a few days off work. That was back in 1987 the last year my life would look "normal" to me.

1988 hit me with a vengeance, my marriage had ended the year before I was about to be remarried it was also the year I heard the words Rheumatoid Arthritis for the first time. It started with a routine visit to my family doctor if you could call her that, you see I rarely saw a doctor back then. I'm the kind of person that waits until a cold turns to Pneumonia before being seen. I think I inherited that trait from my mom I don't remember her ever seeing a doctor until her later years, she hated them.

This particular day I had gone to see her for what I suspected was a sinus infection, I had many previous and to this day still deal with them. She examined me did some routine blood work since it had been so long since my last visit there was nothing out of the ordinary. Before I left she noticed the middle finger on my right hand was swollen and slightly bent, I had been ignoring that fact hoping it would go away since it didn't hurt at that time.

She made some notes, handed me a prescription for the sinus infection, told me when we were heading out the door. "Oh by the way I think you have Rheumatoid Arthritis". I said "what do I do for that?" I mean I had no idea at the time. Back then I associated "Arthritis" with an old peoples disease. She looked back told me "just take an aspirin, you'll be fine" and left the room. I wasn't panicked I thought okay if she isn't worried about it then I shouldn't be either. I couldn't have been more wrong.

Within a week of that visit my wrists had swollen to double their size they were on fire, I was in agony! I hadn't slept in over a week the pain was so bad it felt like I was being stabbed by hot pokers.

I couldn't take it anymore so I made an appointment to see a different general practitioner, he took one look at me and made an appointment for me to see me my first Rheumatologist. I didn't know what to expect for my first visit, I mean back then I was thinking what the heck is a Rheumatologist?

I just wanted to get back to my life! I was young, soft spoken, intimidated, in agony and uneducated as far as RA goes.

I walked into this little cold, uninviting room, sat there alone waiting more than 45 minutes past my appointment time. The Rheumatologist walked in he was as cold as the room I sat in, arrogant, he didn't listen to me and he didn't even exam me! He echoed the aspirin comment and left the room. I had waited 45 minuted for a 5 minute visit.

Within days of that visit I was sitting in a wheelchair in another Rheumatologist's office this one was located in a teaching hospital this experience was totally different the doctor talked to me like a human being, he listened to me, examined me, ordered blood work, then admitted me to the hospital for two weeks. They had a course for new patients with Rheumatoid Arthritis, you went to classes everyday all day as well as getting treatment for the disease. At that time I was getting cortisone through an IV.

They taught me everything I needed to know about Rheumatoid Arthritis. How to live with it, how to exercise, how to modify my home, they had physical therapy classes, occupational therapy classes, they did wax therapy on my hands, made splints for my wrists. I went to the pool every morning for water therapy, I was exhausted but it was the best thing that could have happened to me back then.

From that experience I learned It takes time to develop a good relationship with your doctor, I also learned to stand up for myself. I learned that doctors don't have all the answers and they shouldn't be expected to. Your doctor is an important part of your team so you need to find one you are comfortable with, one who will listen to you and one you will listen to.

I had to change doctor's more times than I can count due to changes in life circumstances. I think I have met every kind of doctor there is from the "it's all in your head" kind to the kind that's just there for the money then there's the "I went to school you know nothing" kind.

My favorite kind was Doctor I know everything, even more than every other Rheumatologist out there! I asked this doctor for a referral to see another Rheumatologist for a second opinion on something, his response to me was "you don't need to go there, he can't do anything I can't do." His attitude completely changed when my husband walked in the room.

Then there are the doctor's who have a bad bedside manner but are great doctors. If you can handle their attitudes you will get great results.

Since my release from the hospital in 1988 I have been on more medications that I can remember. Prednisone in every form that is available, all of the anti inflammatories you can name. Due to GERD and other issues I can no longer take them.

Then came Penicillamine, Plaquenil, Gold shots, Methotrexate pills, Methotrexate injections, all of these medications failed me. You notice I say failed me, I don't believe in saying I failed them I didn't do anything wrong! Then came Arava and Humira, I'm currently working with my doctor to decide what is the next option for me.

My life as I knew it changed in 1988. I was always active I loved to exercise, I walked everywhere it was my form of "therapy." I was always ready to have fun! My friends were always around me, I had a passion for dancing I think I miss that the most.

As I sit here now both of my wrists are surgically fused, they fused on their own after the initial flare in 1988 the onset was swift and the damage was severe. The decision to surgically fuse them was to take away the pain. It worked!

I had a total knee replacement on my right knee in 2010

During the knee replacement the nerve was damaged, people tell me that is a rare complication. That seems to be the story of my life! I had surgery again in 2012 to try and fix the damage. I still have foot drop, it is better than before the surgery but I will never fully recover. My knee still swells and gets sore. I am currently having issues with my feet as well and will require surgery soon.

I had cataract surgery on both eyes a few years ago, I couldn't read the largest letters on the eye chart at the point right before surgery. My optometrist believes it is due to past Prednisone use. Sjogren's Syndrome which accompanies Rheumatoid Arthritis affects my vision, I have trouble seeing due to the extreme dryness in my eyes. The usual treatments haven't worked so far, the next step is punctal plugs in the top and bottom of my eyes. Sjogren's has also caused extensive damage to my teeth as well, I can't be without water for any amount of time sue to extreme dry mouth.

Rheumatoid Arthritis along with the other Autoimmune Arthritis Diseases that accompany it has taken a toll on relationships both personal and professional in my life. I have been unable to work outside the home for the past 12 years. I miss working with people, the connection to the outside world, the ability to make money, I also miss the social aspect.

It is hard to keep the same lifestyle you had before you had RA. Your life is no longer predictable, you don't know when the next flare is coming, how long it will last, if you will be able to move or get out of bed, if you will be able to sleep the night before. I have to plan everything in advance from bathroom stops to where the nearest water is, how many steps there are, how cold or hot the day is going to be, what kind of food there is, how many people will be there, is there a place to sit, how long the event is, half the time I'm not even able to go!

I find it hard meeting new people due to the isolation of these illnesses. Especially when you're at home much of the time and living in an unfamiliar place. When you're exhausted most of the time people don't understand, or sometimes forget about you. There are people in my life who knew me before my illness that stayed with me after. It is important to have a connection with someone and not let this illness completely isolate you. The online world has been a huge source of support for me.

I have connected to others like me through their Blogs, online support groups, Facebook pages, Twitter, and through volunteer work with organizations who deal with Autoimmune Arthritis. if you told me 25 years ago I would meet all these amazing people I would have said you were crazy! I'm thankful for every single one of them.

Since my initial RA diagnosis I have been diagnosed with Sjogren's Syndrome, Raynaud's, Lupus, possible Fibromyalgia, Migraines, GERD, irregular heart rate, just to name a few.

I spend my time these days going to dirt track races in the summer, going on picnics, writing my blog, volunteering with the International Foundation for Autoimmune Arthritis. Going to movies, concerts, taking day trips, spending time with my family and grandchildren, I try to find things I can do and not concentrate on the things I can't do anymore.

After 25+ years of this disease I'm excited to see the advances that have been made. There are more medications than ever for RA as well as other Autoimmune Arthritis Diseases. I believe that had these medications been made available years ago I might not have the damage I do today, it's hard to say. I do know there is hope people are more open to talking, listening and working together to find answers for these diseases.

This is just a small part of my story, it is still being written. I hope in reading this you know you are not alone. There are people fighting for you and with you. To the newly diagnosed I would tell you I know it's scary the most important thing to do is educate yourself, ask questions, find a support system and don't be afraid to stand up for yourself, you are your best advocate. Last but not least it's not your fault!

Tara Manriquez

I was around 11 when it all started. I remember the day clearly two friends and I were riding our bikes, we stopped to pick some wildflowers. I got back on my bike and my knees wouldn't move right, they were stuck slightly bent and I just couldn't get them to move right. I knew I was going down, to this day I remember this all in slow motion I started falling, it seemed like forever before I hit the ground, I caught myself with my right wrist.

Fast forward two years. I'm walking home from the bus stop like I did everyday. My knee doesn't feel right suddenly it wobbles to the side and I fall. I was home, in my own yard, this made me feel safer somehow, even though I couldn't walk. Mum or Dad should be here soon I'll be ok, they'll make it all better right.

All through high school I danced on the Dance Team there were times my knee looked as big as a base ball and times I would collapse, but I was tough I would shake it off and keep going. Often times my hips would move beyond it's normal range I had this swivel thing I would do to try to rotate it back to where it needed to be. If my knee gave out I'd wrap it and dance harder. I never really knew what was going on, but I wasn't going to let it slow me down. Now I know it was a flare of my Juvenile Rheumatoid Arthritis. Luckily throughout my childhood and teen years I also had several disease remission periods, where my disease was quiet and I could forget I had a bad knee and a bad hip.

At 20 I was young married and expecting our first baby, I was working hard so we could save up enough for me to stay home and raise our children. I woke up one morning unable to walk and I had a huge growth on the side of my foot, but I was determined not to miss work so my husband went and got me some crutches and off to work I went. We made an appointment with a doctor and found the growth would have to be removed surgically and that because I was pregnant I would have to be awake for the surgery. The doctor was a very rude arrogant man, but it was a small town and I didn't have a lot of choices. His explanation of the growth was the body does weird things when pregnant, I bought it because he's the doctor and he would know right? I have since learned that what they removed was a rheumatoid nodule.

A few months later I delivered a healthy baby girl. After my daughter was born I would often have days where my body ached and it was hard to get out of bed I just figured its from carrying around a baby my body is not used to these movements. Two years later another little blessing came into our lives, two little girls now to play with. There was plenty of running, chasing, crawling around, ups and downs and my body felt every little movement, but I was happy and love my kids it was all worth it. I loved being home with them and watching every wonder through their eyes for the first time, but found I fatigued very easily.

My husband is a military man. Being at home with the kids was perfect for us while our girls were growing. Often times he would have to be away from us. When the girls got older and were well into their school years my dream job became available and I jumped at the opportunity. I was working with the Special Ed. I always had a soft spot for children and volunteered with the special ed classes all through my school years. This job was perfect for me I would have almost the same hours as my girls were in school for and we would have the same vacation times. It was really a perfect situation for me.

I was lifting children in and out of their wheelchairs and noticed I was getting really sore again. I started to feel I couldn't do it alone and would often have another person lift

with me, I didn't want to hurt the kids. We do a lot of hand over hand for coordination and

fine motor skills and I would notice my hands were swollen and sore, but I'm just using them

more so it's my body adjusting again to new changes. I always worked as a substitute but

would often fill the same position for a long time, subbing worked perfect with my

husband's military career because when he would be away I could take the time off easily

without guilt.

Well it happened he got called to war. He would deploy to Iraq. I felt oddly calm we

knew this day was a possibility, we knew it would come. I let my job go knowing that after

he got home I would go back to work. I had everything lined up, I had contacts for if I

needed different things, the military has everything all prepared should you need help with

anything from a leaky faucet, to help figuring out how to pay your bills. I had a list of

numbers if I needed them, I really felt that I was covered if anything and I mean anything

went wrong.

Technology is an amazing thing if I stayed up late enough I could actually catch my

husband online and although I couldn't see him or hear him we could send emails back and

forth rapidly like we're chatting, maybe more like texting. I was starved to hear from him, he

had no set schedule I just knew he was awake and there maybe an opportunity for us to

chat. I would wait and hope and wait some more often falling asleep at my computer, we

did get to chat often and it was amazing, but never knowing when was not doing well for my

sleep because after staying up all night to get to chat with him for a few minutes I would

have to get up and get the girls off to school, and run the household as the only parent home. Kudos to the single parents who do this all the time. Well I noticed some things happening again my hands are stiff sometimes, painful and swollen others, hot to touch. My hip that used to bother me so often is acting up again. I'm sure that all this is easily explained, I'm typing all hours of the night so of course my hands are angry. I go back and forth between falling asleep on the couch and making it to my bed, I'm sure it's the couch that's bothering my hip.

I start getting fevered and just feel crummy, I think oh no I'm coming down with the flu, I really don't have time for this. I finally broke down and went to my primary physician. I had listed out everything that might be a possible symptom. I must have came in with a pretty good list because right away he asked if I had any family history of autoimmune diseases such as rheumatoid arthritis or lupus; I said I recall my mother saying her Grandfather had rheumatoid arthritis and was no longer able to play his violin, he had been in the London symphony. My primary physician ordered some blood tests and gave me a referral to see a rheumatologist, the type of dr that deals with rheumatic autoimmune diseases.

I found a local Rheumatologist who was really at the top of this field, world renowned and highly recommended. I made an appt. he first tells me I have fibromyalgia, the only things I knew about this were rumors that it's diagnosed when drs don't know what's going on. I didn't understand I was first meeting him and he's already blowing me off. He does let me know I had some blood work that came back with some questions he wanted answered he wanted more blood work done and X-rays for good measure. The other thing he did was start me on physical therapy. He works closely with one physical therapist that can watch for different symptoms and then they would meet weekly and compare notes, its this method that he used that helped him diagnose me so quickly. Between the high inflammation rates in my blood and the swelling the physical therapist had seen, plus appointments with the Dr. I was quickly diagnosed with Rheumatoid arthritis, mixed tissue disease, and raynads syndrome. It was a lot to swallow. I put on a brave face and thanked him telling him I would think about the medication options which really scared me; shots, infusions, immune suppressants, chemo drugs. My head was spinning I didn't know whether to cry or throw up.

I went straight from the doctor to my husband, (who had recently returned home safe and sound) and I broke down. He was asking questions I didn't have answers to. Just give me this moment to feel sad and hold me.

Then I went to work educating myself. I found the local arthritis foundation was having a walk, I would go and gobble up all the information I could. At the walk there were drug manufacturers pamphlets, DVDs and information galore. I researched them all and chose what I thought would be best for me. Since then I have been through 4 different DMARDs (disease modifying anti rheumatic drugs) and 5 biologics. Biologics are the new go to medication for autoimmune arthritis diseases, they are hoped to slow the disease progress and are all either given via an injection or an IV infusion. For many of us these meds aren't working and when one does work it can fail after a while. That is the problem I am having.

Right now I am on monthly infusions which are given in a small infusion room with no windows and no art on the walls. It is really a depressing room the lv poles are outdated and don't have monitors on them. My husband comes with me to every appointment, but is not allowed to come into the infusion room with me. The medications are extremely expensive I am very lucky my insurance covers them.

My hope is that there will be more awareness brought to these diseases, which will lead to better funding for better research and new medications. I like many others try to advocate and educate people to raise awareness, which we hope will help raise more funds for better research and better medications.

I am only 38 years old I walk more like an 80 year old. I have both a manual and an electric wheelchair that enables me to do things with my family like taking a trip to the zoo. Without the chair there is no way I could physically walk that far anymore, at least not without paying for it later with severe pain and fatigue.

I'm learning to do things in a whole new way. I have the love, support, and understanding of my family. These are the important things in life. I've had to slow down a lot and can't do a lot of the things I used to love to do, but you know what I have more time to watch the wild critters outside my window, time to read more, time to relax on my porch swing and if I'm quiet enough the birds will approach me. Time to watch sappy movies with my family and to prove to my daughters the 80s really were the best at making love stories. I have always loved the little things like barefoot walks on a cool summer evening.

My disease has also opened up more worlds to me especially online. I have made some amazing friends through online support groups. I have started my own blog to share my experience with others and to make more connections to new friends. My life has changed, but it's still wonderful and full of love laughter and beauty. Now I have more time to pay attention to the special moments, and guess what they are all special. I have lost many friends to this disease it really reminds me to savor every moment because you never know when things will change.

On a separate note my oldest daughter is the one who came up with this Anthology as a way to raise awareness and to let our voice be heard. She's 17 now and already a published author. She is an amazing daughter and makes me so proud. I hope you enjoy our stories.